This Book Belongs To:

Contact Information	
Name:	
Phone:	
Email:	

Start / End Date

/ / to / /

Dedication

This book is dedicated to all the exercisers around the world, who strive every day to bring their "A" game and create the body and life they desire.

You are my inspiration for producing books and I'm excited to help people keep track of their fitness goals and progress – together, we can make the world a happier and healthier place!

How to Use This Fitness Tracker

This ultimate fitness tracker will help anyone reach their fitness goals by offering a comprehensive way to keep track of each exercise, whether you're focused on strength training, cardio, improved diet, or any other goals – you can make progress when you use this tracker daily.

Here are some simple guidelines to follow so you can get the most out of this book:

1. The first section features boxes where you can fill in the Date, Time, Weight, Body Fat, Muscle Group, Warm Up and Stretch. This is a great snapshot of each day, and it will make it very clear which areas you need to work on next.

2. The next section is all about strength training. More and more research has shown that strength training is important for every person. You can list the workout you performed, the sets, reps, and weight used. This is handy to flip back and see what weight you were the last time you did the exercise, so you can keep making progress and not guess.

3. The third section is where you can track your cardio. Featuring which Exercise, Duration, Distance, Calories, and Heart Rate, you can confidently make strides in cardio by jotting down this information during rests.

4. The last section features Notes/Nutrition, and rating your Body Strength and Mind Power. This is a great place to see how the rest of your life is affecting your physical health – and you can make notes of anything that comes to mind. You may begin to see patterns emerge about your health. Knowledge is power.

📅 **DATE**		⏱️ **TIME**	
⚖️ **WEIGHT**		📏 **BODY FAT**	
💪 **MUSCLE GROUP**		☐ **WARM-UP**	☐ **STRETCH**

🏋️ **STRENGTH TRAINING**			SET 1	SET 1	SET 1	SET 1	SET 1	SET 1
EXERCISE		REPS						
		WEIGHT						
		REPS						
		WEIGHT						
		REPS						
		WEIGHT						
		REPS						
		WEIGHT						
		REPS						
		WEIGHT						
		REPS						
		WEIGHT						
		REPS						
		WEIGHT						
		REPS						
		WEIGHT						

👟 **CARDIO**		DURATION	DISTANCE	CALORIES	HEART RATE
EXERCISE					

NOTES / NUTRITION

RATING	
⚡ BODY STRENGTH	☆☆☆☆☆
🧠 MIND POWER	☆☆☆☆☆

📅 **DATE**		⏱️ **TIME**	
⚖️ **WEIGHT**		📏 **BODY FAT**	
💪 **MUSCLE GROUP**		☐ **WARM-UP**	☐ **STRETCH**

🏋️ STRENGTH TRAINING

EXERCISE			SET 1	SET 1	SET 1	SET 1	SET 1	SET 1
		REPS						
		WEIGHT						
		REPS						
		WEIGHT						
		REPS						
		WEIGHT						
		REPS						
		WEIGHT						
		REPS						
		WEIGHT						
		REPS						
		WEIGHT						
		REPS						
		WEIGHT						
		REPS						
		WEIGHT						

👟 CARDIO

EXERCISE		DURATION	DISTANCE	CALORIES	HEART RATE

NOTES / NUTRITION	**RATING**	
	⚡ BODY STRENGTH	☆☆☆☆☆
	🧠 MIND POWER	☆☆☆☆☆

📅 DATE		⏱️ TIME	
⚖️ WEIGHT		📏 BODY FAT	
💪 MUSCLE GROUP		☐ WARM-UP	☐ STRETCH

🏋️ STRENGTH TRAINING

EXERCISE			SET 1	SET 1	SET 1	SET 1	SET 1	SET 1
		REPS						
		WEIGHT						
		REPS						
		WEIGHT						
		REPS						
		WEIGHT						
		REPS						
		WEIGHT						
		REPS						
		WEIGHT						
		REPS						
		WEIGHT						
		REPS						
		WEIGHT						
		REPS						
		WEIGHT						

👟 CARDIO

EXERCISE		DURATION	DISTANCE	CALORIES	HEART RATE

NOTES / NUTRITION

RATING

⚡ BODY STRENGTH	☆☆☆☆☆
🧠 MIND POWER	☆☆☆☆☆

📅 DATE		🕐 TIME	
⚖️ WEIGHT		📏 BODY FAT	
💪 MUSCLE GROUP		☐ WARM-UP	☐ STRETCH

🏋️ STRENGTH TRAINING

EXERCISE			SET 1	SET 1	SET 1	SET 1	SET 1	SET 1
		REPS						
		WEIGHT						
		REPS						
		WEIGHT						
		REPS						
		WEIGHT						
		REPS						
		WEIGHT						
		REPS						
		WEIGHT						
		REPS						
		WEIGHT						
		REPS						
		WEIGHT						
		REPS						
		WEIGHT						

👟 CARDIO

EXERCISE		DURATION	DISTANCE	CALORIES	HEART RATE

NOTES / NUTRITION

RATING

⚡ BODY STRENGTH	☆☆☆☆☆
🧠 MIND POWER	☆☆☆☆☆

📅 DATE		⏱ TIME	
⚖ WEIGHT		📏 BODY FAT	
💪 MUSCLE GROUP		☐ WARM-UP	☐ STRETCH

🏋 STRENGTH TRAINING

EXERCISE			SET 1	SET 1	SET 1	SET 1	SET 1	SET 1
		REPS						
		WEIGHT						
		REPS						
		WEIGHT						
		REPS						
		WEIGHT						
		REPS						
		WEIGHT						
		REPS						
		WEIGHT						
		REPS						
		WEIGHT						
		REPS						
		WEIGHT						
		REPS						
		WEIGHT						

👟 CARDIO

EXERCISE		DURATION	DISTANCE	CALORIES	HEART RATE

NOTES / NUTRITION	RATING
	⚡ BODY STRENGTH ☆☆☆☆☆
	🧠 MIND POWER ☆☆☆☆☆

📅 DATE		⏱️ TIME	
⚖️ WEIGHT		📏 BODY FAT	
💪 MUSCLE GROUP		☐ WARM-UP	☐ STRETCH

🏋️ STRENGTH TRAINING

EXERCISE			SET 1	SET 1	SET 1	SET 1	SET 1	SET 1
		REPS						
		WEIGHT						
		REPS						
		WEIGHT						
		REPS						
		WEIGHT						
		REPS						
		WEIGHT						
		REPS						
		WEIGHT						
		REPS						
		WEIGHT						
		REPS						
		WEIGHT						
		REPS						
		WEIGHT						

👟 CARDIO

EXERCISE		DURATION	DISTANCE	CALORIES	HEART RATE

NOTES / NUTRITION

RATING

⚡	BODY STRENGTH	☆☆☆☆☆
🧠	MIND POWER	☆☆☆☆☆

📅 DATE		🕐 TIME	
⚖ WEIGHT		📏 BODY FAT	
💪 MUSCLE GROUP		☐ WARM-UP	☐ STRETCH

🏋 STRENGTH TRAINING			SET 1	SET 1	SET 1	SET 1	SET 1	SET 1
EXERCISE		REPS						
		WEIGHT						
		REPS						
		WEIGHT						
		REPS						
		WEIGHT						
		REPS						
		WEIGHT						
		REPS						
		WEIGHT						
		REPS						
		WEIGHT						
		REPS						
		WEIGHT						
		REPS						
		WEIGHT						

👟 CARDIO		DURATION	DISTANCE	CALORIES	HEART RATE
EXERCISE					

NOTES / NUTRITION

RATING	
⚡ BODY STRENGTH	☆☆☆☆☆
🧠 MIND POWER	☆☆☆☆☆

	DATE		TIME
	WEIGHT		BODY FAT
	MUSCLE GROUP		☐ WARM-UP ☐ STRETCH

STRENGTH TRAINING

EXERCISE			SET 1	SET 1	SET 1	SET 1	SET 1	SET 1
		REPS						
		WEIGHT						
		REPS						
		WEIGHT						
		REPS						
		WEIGHT						
		REPS						
		WEIGHT						
		REPS						
		WEIGHT						
		REPS						
		WEIGHT						
		REPS						
		WEIGHT						
		REPS						
		WEIGHT						

CARDIO

EXERCISE		DURATION	DISTANCE	CALORIES	HEART RATE

NOTES / NUTRITION

RATING

	BODY STRENGTH	☆☆☆☆☆
	MIND POWER	☆☆☆☆☆

📅 DATE		⏱ TIME	
🛁 WEIGHT		📏 BODY FAT	
💪 MUSCLE GROUP		☐ WARM-UP	☐ STRETCH

🏋 STRENGTH TRAINING

			SET 1	SET 1	SET 1	SET 1	SET 1	SET 1
E X E R C I S E		REPS						
		WEIGHT						
		REPS						
		WEIGHT						
		REPS						
		WEIGHT						
		REPS						
		WEIGHT						
		REPS						
		WEIGHT						
		REPS						
		WEIGHT						
		REPS						
		WEIGHT						
		REPS						
		WEIGHT						

👟 CARDIO

		DURATION	DISTANCE	CALORIES	HEART RATE
E X E R C I S E					

NOTES / NUTRITION	RATING
	⚡ BODY STRENGTH ☆☆☆☆☆
	🧠 MIND POWER ☆☆☆☆☆

	DATE			TIME	
	WEIGHT			BODY FAT	
	MUSCLE GROUP		☐ WARM-UP	☐ STRETCH	

STRENGTH TRAINING

			SET 1	SET 1	SET 1	SET 1	SET 1	SET 1
EXERCISE		REPS						
		WEIGHT						
		REPS						
		WEIGHT						
		REPS						
		WEIGHT						
		REPS						
		WEIGHT						
		REPS						
		WEIGHT						
		REPS						
		WEIGHT						
		REPS						
		WEIGHT						
		REPS						
		WEIGHT						

CARDIO

		DURATION	DISTANCE	CALORIES	HEART RATE
EXERCISE					

NOTES / NUTRITION

RATING

⚡	BODY STRENGTH	☆☆☆☆☆
🧠	MIND POWER	☆☆☆☆☆

📅 DATE		🕐 TIME	
⚖️ WEIGHT		📏 BODY FAT	
💪 MUSCLE GROUP		☐ WARM-UP	☐ STRETCH

🏋️ STRENGTH TRAINING

EXERCISE			SET 1	SET 1	SET 1	SET 1	SET 1	SET 1
		REPS						
		WEIGHT						
		REPS						
		WEIGHT						
		REPS						
		WEIGHT						
		REPS						
		WEIGHT						
		REPS						
		WEIGHT						
		REPS						
		WEIGHT						
		REPS						
		WEIGHT						
		REPS						
		WEIGHT						

👟 CARDIO

EXERCISE		DURATION	DISTANCE	CALORIES	HEART RATE

NOTES / NUTRITION	RATING	
	⚡ BODY STRENGTH	☆☆☆☆☆
	🧠 MIND POWER	☆☆☆☆☆

📅 DATE		🕐 TIME	
⚖️ WEIGHT		📏 BODY FAT	
💪 MUSCLE GROUP		☐ WARM-UP	☐ STRETCH

🏋️ STRENGTH TRAINING

EXERCISE			SET 1	SET 1	SET 1	SET 1	SET 1	SET 1
		REPS						
		WEIGHT						
		REPS						
		WEIGHT						
		REPS						
		WEIGHT						
		REPS						
		WEIGHT						
		REPS						
		WEIGHT						
		REPS						
		WEIGHT						
		REPS						
		WEIGHT						
		REPS						
		WEIGHT						

👟 CARDIO

EXERCISE		DURATION	DISTANCE	CALORIES	HEART RATE

NOTES / NUTRITION	RATING
	⚡ BODY STRENGTH ☆☆☆☆☆
	🧠 MIND POWER ☆☆☆☆☆

📅 DATE	⏱️ TIME
⬛ WEIGHT	📏 BODY FAT
💪 MUSCLE GROUP	☐ WARM-UP ☐ STRETCH

🏋️ STRENGTH TRAINING

EXERCISE			SET 1	SET 1	SET 1	SET 1	SET 1	SET 1
		REPS						
		WEIGHT						
		REPS						
		WEIGHT						
		REPS						
		WEIGHT						
		REPS						
		WEIGHT						
		REPS						
		WEIGHT						
		REPS						
		WEIGHT						
		REPS						
		WEIGHT						
		REPS						
		WEIGHT						

👟 CARDIO

EXERCISE		DURATION	DISTANCE	CALORIES	HEART RATE

NOTES / NUTRITION	RATING
	⚡ BODY STRENGTH ☆☆☆☆☆
	🧠 MIND POWER ☆☆☆☆☆

📅 DATE		⏱️ TIME	
⚖️ WEIGHT		📏 BODY FAT	
💪 MUSCLE GROUP		☐ WARM-UP	☐ STRETCH

🏋️ STRENGTH TRAINING

EXERCISE			SET 1	SET 1	SET 1	SET 1	SET 1	SET 1
		REPS						
		WEIGHT						
		REPS						
		WEIGHT						
		REPS						
		WEIGHT						
		REPS						
		WEIGHT						
		REPS						
		WEIGHT						
		REPS						
		WEIGHT						
		REPS						
		WEIGHT						
		REPS						
		WEIGHT						

👟 CARDIO

EXERCISE		DURATION	DISTANCE	CALORIES	HEART RATE

NOTES / NUTRITION	RATING
	⚡ BODY STRENGTH ☆☆☆☆☆
	🧠 MIND POWER ☆☆☆☆☆

📅 DATE		⏱ TIME	
⚖ WEIGHT		📏 BODY FAT	
💪 MUSCLE GROUP		☐ WARM-UP	☐ STRETCH

🏋 STRENGTH TRAINING

EXERCISE			SET 1	SET 1	SET 1	SET 1	SET 1	SET 1
		REPS						
		WEIGHT						
		REPS						
		WEIGHT						
		REPS						
		WEIGHT						
		REPS						
		WEIGHT						
		REPS						
		WEIGHT						
		REPS						
		WEIGHT						
		REPS						
		WEIGHT						
		REPS						
		WEIGHT						

👟 CARDIO

EXERCISE		DURATION	DISTANCE	CALORIES	HEART RATE

NOTES / NUTRITION

RATING

⚡ BODY STRENGTH	☆☆☆☆☆
🧠 MIND POWER	☆☆☆☆☆

📅 DATE		⏱ TIME	
⚖ WEIGHT		📏 BODY FAT	
💪 MUSCLE GROUP		☐ WARM-UP	☐ STRETCH

🏋 STRENGTH TRAINING

EXERCISE			SET 1	SET 1	SET 1	SET 1	SET 1	SET 1
		REPS						
		WEIGHT						
		REPS						
		WEIGHT						
		REPS						
		WEIGHT						
		REPS						
		WEIGHT						
		REPS						
		WEIGHT						
		REPS						
		WEIGHT						
		REPS						
		WEIGHT						
		REPS						
		WEIGHT						

👟 CARDIO

EXERCISE		DURATION	DISTANCE	CALORIES	HEART RATE

NOTES / NUTRITION	RATING	
	⚡ BODY STRENGTH	☆☆☆☆☆
	🧠 MIND POWER	☆☆☆☆☆

	DATE		TIME
	WEIGHT		BODY FAT
	MUSCLE GROUP	☐ WARM-UP	☐ STRETCH

STRENGTH TRAINING

EXERCISE			SET 1	SET 1	SET 1	SET 1	SET 1	SET 1
		REPS						
		WEIGHT						
		REPS						
		WEIGHT						
		REPS						
		WEIGHT						
		REPS						
		WEIGHT						
		REPS						
		WEIGHT						
		REPS						
		WEIGHT						
		REPS						
		WEIGHT						
		REPS						
		WEIGHT						

CARDIO

EXERCISE		DURATION	DISTANCE	CALORIES	HEART RATE

NOTES / NUTRITION	RATING	
	BODY STRENGTH	☆☆☆☆☆
	MIND POWER	☆☆☆☆☆

📅 DATE		⏱ TIME	
⚖ WEIGHT		📏 BODY FAT	
💪 MUSCLE GROUP		☐ WARM-UP	☐ STRETCH

🏋 STRENGTH TRAINING

EXERCISE			SET 1	SET 1	SET 1	SET 1	SET 1	SET 1
		REPS						
		WEIGHT						
		REPS						
		WEIGHT						
		REPS						
		WEIGHT						
		REPS						
		WEIGHT						
		REPS						
		WEIGHT						
		REPS						
		WEIGHT						
		REPS						
		WEIGHT						
		REPS						
		WEIGHT						

👟 CARDIO

EXERCISE		DURATION	DISTANCE	CALORIES	HEART RATE

NOTES / NUTRITION

RATING

⚡ BODY STRENGTH	☆☆☆☆☆
🧠 MIND POWER	☆☆☆☆☆

📅 DATE		🕐 TIME	
⚖️ WEIGHT		🧵 BODY FAT	
💪 MUSCLE GROUP		☐ WARM-UP	☐ STRETCH

🏋️ STRENGTH TRAINING

EXERCISE			SET 1	SET 1	SET 1	SET 1	SET 1	SET 1
		REPS						
		WEIGHT						
		REPS						
		WEIGHT						
		REPS						
		WEIGHT						
		REPS						
		WEIGHT						
		REPS						
		WEIGHT						
		REPS						
		WEIGHT						
		REPS						
		WEIGHT						
		REPS						
		WEIGHT						

👟 CARDIO

EXERCISE	DURATION	DISTANCE	CALORIES	HEART RATE

NOTES / NUTRITION

RATING

⚡ BODY STRENGTH	☆☆☆☆☆
🧠 MIND POWER	☆☆☆☆☆

📅 DATE		🕐 TIME	
⚖️ WEIGHT		📏 BODY FAT	
💪 MUSCLE GROUP		☐ WARM-UP	☐ STRETCH

🏋️ STRENGTH TRAINING

EXERCISE			SET 1	SET 1	SET 1	SET 1	SET 1	SET 1
		REPS						
		WEIGHT						
		REPS						
		WEIGHT						
		REPS						
		WEIGHT						
		REPS						
		WEIGHT						
		REPS						
		WEIGHT						
		REPS						
		WEIGHT						
		REPS						
		WEIGHT						
		REPS						
		WEIGHT						

👟 CARDIO

EXERCISE		DURATION	DISTANCE	CALORIES	HEART RATE

NOTES / NUTRITION

RATING

⚡ BODY STRENGTH	☆☆☆☆☆
🧠 MIND POWER	☆☆☆☆☆

	DATE		TIME
	WEIGHT		BODY FAT
	MUSCLE GROUP	☐ WARM-UP	☐ STRETCH

STRENGTH TRAINING

EXERCISE			SET 1	SET 1	SET 1	SET 1	SET 1	SET 1
		REPS						
		WEIGHT						
		REPS						
		WEIGHT						
		REPS						
		WEIGHT						
		REPS						
		WEIGHT						
		REPS						
		WEIGHT						
		REPS						
		WEIGHT						
		REPS						
		WEIGHT						
		REPS						
		WEIGHT						

CARDIO

EXERCISE		DURATION	DISTANCE	CALORIES	HEART RATE

NOTES / NUTRITION

RATING

⚡	BODY STRENGTH	☆☆☆☆☆
🧠	MIND POWER	☆☆☆☆☆

📅 DATE		🕐 TIME	
⚖️ WEIGHT		📏 BODY FAT	
💪 MUSCLE GROUP		☐ WARM-UP	☐ STRETCH

🏋️ STRENGTH TRAINING

EXERCISE			SET 1	SET 1	SET 1	SET 1	SET 1	SET 1
		REPS						
		WEIGHT						
		REPS						
		WEIGHT						
		REPS						
		WEIGHT						
		REPS						
		WEIGHT						
		REPS						
		WEIGHT						
		REPS						
		WEIGHT						
		REPS						
		WEIGHT						
		REPS						
		WEIGHT						

👟 CARDIO

EXERCISE		DURATION	DISTANCE	CALORIES	HEART RATE

NOTES / NUTRITION

RATING

⚡ BODY STRENGTH	☆☆☆☆☆
🧠 MIND POWER	☆☆☆☆☆

📅 DATE		🕐 TIME	
⚖️ WEIGHT		📏 BODY FAT	
💪 MUSCLE GROUP		☐ WARM-UP	☐ STRETCH

🏋️ STRENGTH TRAINING			SET 1	SET 1	SET 1	SET 1	SET 1	SET 1
E X E R C I S E		REPS						
		WEIGHT						
		REPS						
		WEIGHT						
		REPS						
		WEIGHT						
		REPS						
		WEIGHT						
		REPS						
		WEIGHT						
		REPS						
		WEIGHT						
		REPS						
		WEIGHT						
		REPS						
		WEIGHT						

👟 CARDIO		DURATION	DISTANCE	CALORIES	HEART RATE
E X E R C I S E					

NOTES / NUTRITION

RATING	
⚡ BODY STRENGTH	☆☆☆☆☆
🧠 MIND POWER	☆☆☆☆☆

📅 DATE		⏱️ TIME	
⚖️ WEIGHT		📏 BODY FAT	
💪 MUSCLE GROUP		☐ WARM-UP	☐ STRETCH

🏋️ STRENGTH TRAINING			SET 1	SET 1	SET 1	SET 1	SET 1	SET 1
EXERCISE		REPS						
		WEIGHT						
		REPS						
		WEIGHT						
		REPS						
		WEIGHT						
		REPS						
		WEIGHT						
		REPS						
		WEIGHT						
		REPS						
		WEIGHT						
		REPS						
		WEIGHT						
		REPS						
		WEIGHT						

👟 CARDIO		DURATION	DISTANCE	CALORIES	HEART RATE
EXERCISE					

NOTES / NUTRITION

RATING	
⚡ BODY STRENGTH	☆☆☆☆☆
🧠 MIND POWER	☆☆☆☆☆

📅 DATE		⏱️ TIME	
🖼️ WEIGHT		📏 BODY FAT	
💪 MUSCLE GROUP		☐ WARM-UP	☐ STRETCH

🏋️ STRENGTH TRAINING

EXERCISE			SET 1	SET 1	SET 1	SET 1	SET 1	SET 1
		REPS						
		WEIGHT						
		REPS						
		WEIGHT						
		REPS						
		WEIGHT						
		REPS						
		WEIGHT						
		REPS						
		WEIGHT						
		REPS						
		WEIGHT						
		REPS						
		WEIGHT						
		REPS						
		WEIGHT						

👟 CARDIO

EXERCISE	DURATION	DISTANCE	CALORIES	HEART RATE

NOTES / NUTRITION

RATING

⚡ BODY STRENGTH	☆☆☆☆☆
🧠 MIND POWER	☆☆☆☆☆

📅 DATE		⏱️ TIME	
⚖️ WEIGHT		📏 BODY FAT	
💪 MUSCLE GROUP		☐ WARM-UP	☐ STRETCH

🏋️ STRENGTH TRAINING

EXERCISE			SET 1	SET 1	SET 1	SET 1	SET 1	SET 1
		REPS						
		WEIGHT						
		REPS						
		WEIGHT						
		REPS						
		WEIGHT						
		REPS						
		WEIGHT						
		REPS						
		WEIGHT						
		REPS						
		WEIGHT						
		REPS						
		WEIGHT						
		REPS						
		WEIGHT						

👟 CARDIO

EXERCISE	DURATION	DISTANCE	CALORIES	HEART RATE

NOTES / NUTRITION	RATING	
	⚡ BODY STRENGTH	☆☆☆☆☆
	🧠 MIND POWER	☆☆☆☆☆

📅 DATE		⏱️ TIME	
⚖️ WEIGHT		📏 BODY FAT	
💪 MUSCLE GROUP		☐ WARM-UP	☐ STRETCH

🏋️ STRENGTH TRAINING			SET 1	SET 1	SET 1	SET 1	SET 1	SET 1
E X E R C I S E		REPS						
		WEIGHT						
		REPS						
		WEIGHT						
		REPS						
		WEIGHT						
		REPS						
		WEIGHT						
		REPS						
		WEIGHT						
		REPS						
		WEIGHT						
		REPS						
		WEIGHT						
		REPS						
		WEIGHT						

👟 CARDIO		DURATION	DISTANCE	CALORIES	HEART RATE
E X E R C I S E					

NOTES / NUTRITION

RATING	
⚡ BODY STRENGTH	☆☆☆☆☆
🧠 MIND POWER	☆☆☆☆☆

📅 DATE		⏱️ TIME	
⚖️ WEIGHT		📏 BODY FAT	
💪 MUSCLE GROUP		☐ WARM-UP	☐ STRETCH

🏋️ STRENGTH TRAINING

EXERCISE			SET 1	SET 1	SET 1	SET 1	SET 1	SET 1
		REPS						
		WEIGHT						
		REPS						
		WEIGHT						
		REPS						
		WEIGHT						
		REPS						
		WEIGHT						
		REPS						
		WEIGHT						
		REPS						
		WEIGHT						
		REPS						
		WEIGHT						
		REPS						
		WEIGHT						

👟 CARDIO

EXERCISE		DURATION	DISTANCE	CALORIES	HEART RATE

NOTES / NUTRITION

RATING

⚡ BODY STRENGTH	☆☆☆☆☆
🧠 MIND POWER	☆☆☆☆☆

📅 DATE		⏱ TIME
⚖ WEIGHT		📏 BODY FAT
💪 MUSCLE GROUP		☐ WARM-UP ☐ STRETCH

🏋 STRENGTH TRAINING			SET 1	SET 1	SET 1	SET 1	SET 1	SET 1
EXERCISE		REPS						
		WEIGHT						
		REPS						
		WEIGHT						
		REPS						
		WEIGHT						
		REPS						
		WEIGHT						
		REPS						
		WEIGHT						
		REPS						
		WEIGHT						
		REPS						
		WEIGHT						
		REPS						
		WEIGHT						

👟 CARDIO		DURATION	DISTANCE	CALORIES	HEART RATE
EXERCISE					

NOTES / NUTRITION

RATING	
⚡ BODY STRENGTH	☆☆☆☆☆
🧠 MIND POWER	☆☆☆☆☆

📅 DATE		⏱ TIME	
⚖ WEIGHT		📏 BODY FAT	
💪 MUSCLE GROUP		☐ WARM-UP	☐ STRETCH

🏋 STRENGTH TRAINING

EXERCISE			SET 1	SET 1	SET 1	SET 1	SET 1	SET 1
		REPS						
		WEIGHT						
		REPS						
		WEIGHT						
		REPS						
		WEIGHT						
		REPS						
		WEIGHT						
		REPS						
		WEIGHT						
		REPS						
		WEIGHT						
		REPS						
		WEIGHT						
		REPS						
		WEIGHT						

👟 CARDIO

EXERCISE		DURATION	DISTANCE	CALORIES	HEART RATE

NOTES / NUTRITION	RATING		
	⚡ BODY STRENGTH	☆☆☆☆☆	
	🧠 MIND POWER	☆☆☆☆☆	

📅 DATE		⏱ TIME	
⚖ WEIGHT		📏 BODY FAT	
💪 MUSCLE GROUP		☐ WARM-UP	☐ STRETCH

🏋 STRENGTH TRAINING			SET 1	SET 1	SET 1	SET 1	SET 1	SET 1
E X E R C I S E		REPS						
		WEIGHT						
		REPS						
		WEIGHT						
		REPS						
		WEIGHT						
		REPS						
		WEIGHT						
		REPS						
		WEIGHT						
		REPS						
		WEIGHT						
		REPS						
		WEIGHT						
		REPS						
		WEIGHT						

👟 CARDIO		DURATION	DISTANCE	CALORIES	HEART RATE
E X E R C I S E					

NOTES / NUTRITION

RATING	
⚡ BODY STRENGTH	☆☆☆☆☆
🧠 MIND POWER	☆☆☆☆☆

📅 DATE		⏱️ TIME	
⬛ WEIGHT		📏 BODY FAT	
💪 MUSCLE GROUP		☐ WARM-UP	☐ STRETCH

🏋️ STRENGTH TRAINING

EXERCISE			SET 1	SET 1	SET 1	SET 1	SET 1	SET 1
		REPS						
		WEIGHT						
		REPS						
		WEIGHT						
		REPS						
		WEIGHT						
		REPS						
		WEIGHT						
		REPS						
		WEIGHT						
		REPS						
		WEIGHT						
		REPS						
		WEIGHT						
		REPS						
		WEIGHT						

👟 CARDIO

EXERCISE	DURATION	DISTANCE	CALORIES	HEART RATE

NOTES / NUTRITION

RATING	
⚡ BODY STRENGTH	☆☆☆☆☆
🧠 MIND POWER	☆☆☆☆☆

📅 DATE		⏱ TIME	
⚖ WEIGHT		📏 BODY FAT	
💪 MUSCLE GROUP		☐ WARM-UP	☐ STRETCH

🏋 STRENGTH TRAINING

			SET 1	SET 1	SET 1	SET 1	SET 1	SET 1
EXERCISE		REPS						
		WEIGHT						
		REPS						
		WEIGHT						
		REPS						
		WEIGHT						
		REPS						
		WEIGHT						
		REPS						
		WEIGHT						
		REPS						
		WEIGHT						
		REPS						
		WEIGHT						
		REPS						
		WEIGHT						

👟 CARDIO

		DURATION	DISTANCE	CALORIES	HEART RATE
EXERCISE					

NOTES / NUTRITION	RATING	
	⚡ BODY STRENGTH	☆☆☆☆☆
	🧠 MIND POWER	☆☆☆☆☆

📅 DATE		⏱ TIME	
⚖ WEIGHT		📏 BODY FAT	
💪 MUSCLE GROUP		☐ WARM-UP	☐ STRETCH

🏋 STRENGTH TRAINING

EXERCISE			SET 1	SET 1	SET 1	SET 1	SET 1	SET 1
		REPS						
		WEIGHT						
		REPS						
		WEIGHT						
		REPS						
		WEIGHT						
		REPS						
		WEIGHT						
		REPS						
		WEIGHT						
		REPS						
		WEIGHT						
		REPS						
		WEIGHT						
		REPS						
		WEIGHT						

👟 CARDIO

EXERCISE	DURATION	DISTANCE	CALORIES	HEART RATE

NOTES / NUTRITION	RATING	
	⚡ BODY STRENGTH	☆☆☆☆☆
	🧠 MIND POWER	☆☆☆☆☆

📅 DATE		⏱ TIME	
⚖ WEIGHT		📏 BODY FAT	
💪 MUSCLE GROUP		☐ WARM-UP	☐ STRETCH

🏋 STRENGTH TRAINING

EXERCISE			SET 1	SET 1	SET 1	SET 1	SET 1	SET 1
		REPS						
		WEIGHT						
		REPS						
		WEIGHT						
		REPS						
		WEIGHT						
		REPS						
		WEIGHT						
		REPS						
		WEIGHT						
		REPS						
		WEIGHT						
		REPS						
		WEIGHT						
		REPS						
		WEIGHT						

👟 CARDIO

EXERCISE		DURATION	DISTANCE	CALORIES	HEART RATE

NOTES / NUTRITION

RATING

⚡ BODY STRENGTH	☆☆☆☆☆
🧠 MIND POWER	☆☆☆☆☆

📅 DATE		⏱️ TIME	
⚖️ WEIGHT		📏 BODY FAT	
💪 MUSCLE GROUP		☐ WARM-UP	☐ STRETCH

🏋️ STRENGTH TRAINING

EXERCISE			SET 1	SET 1	SET 1	SET 1	SET 1	SET 1
		REPS						
		WEIGHT						
		REPS						
		WEIGHT						
		REPS						
		WEIGHT						
		REPS						
		WEIGHT						
		REPS						
		WEIGHT						
		REPS						
		WEIGHT						
		REPS						
		WEIGHT						
		REPS						
		WEIGHT						

👟 CARDIO

EXERCISE		DURATION	DISTANCE	CALORIES	HEART RATE

NOTES / NUTRITION

RATING

⚡ BODY STRENGTH	☆☆☆☆☆
🧠 MIND POWER	☆☆☆☆☆

📅 DATE		🕐 TIME	
⬛ WEIGHT		📏 BODY FAT	
💪 MUSCLE GROUP		☐ WARM-UP	☐ STRETCH

🏋️ STRENGTH TRAINING

EXERCISE			SET 1	SET 1	SET 1	SET 1	SET 1	SET 1
		REPS						
		WEIGHT						
		REPS						
		WEIGHT						
		REPS						
		WEIGHT						
		REPS						
		WEIGHT						
		REPS						
		WEIGHT						
		REPS						
		WEIGHT						
		REPS						
		WEIGHT						
		REPS						
		WEIGHT						

👟 CARDIO

EXERCISE		DURATION	DISTANCE	CALORIES	HEART RATE

NOTES / NUTRITION

RATING

⚡ BODY STRENGTH	☆☆☆☆☆
🧠 MIND POWER	☆☆☆☆☆

📅 DATE		⏱️ TIME	
⚖️ WEIGHT		📏 BODY FAT	
💪 MUSCLE GROUP		☐ WARM-UP	☐ STRETCH

🏋️ STRENGTH TRAINING

EXERCISE			SET 1	SET 1	SET 1	SET 1	SET 1	SET 1
		REPS						
		WEIGHT						
		REPS						
		WEIGHT						
		REPS						
		WEIGHT						
		REPS						
		WEIGHT						
		REPS						
		WEIGHT						
		REPS						
		WEIGHT						
		REPS						
		WEIGHT						
		REPS						
		WEIGHT						

👟 CARDIO

EXERCISE		DURATION	DISTANCE	CALORIES	HEART RATE

NOTES / NUTRITION

RATING

⚡ BODY STRENGTH	☆☆☆☆☆
🧠 MIND POWER	☆☆☆☆☆

📅 DATE		⏱️ TIME	
🔲 WEIGHT		📏 BODY FAT	
💪 MUSCLE GROUP		☐ WARM-UP	☐ STRETCH

🏋️ STRENGTH TRAINING

EXERCISE			SET 1	SET 1	SET 1	SET 1	SET 1	SET 1
		REPS						
		WEIGHT						
		REPS						
		WEIGHT						
		REPS						
		WEIGHT						
		REPS						
		WEIGHT						
		REPS						
		WEIGHT						
		REPS						
		WEIGHT						
		REPS						
		WEIGHT						
		REPS						
		WEIGHT						

👟 CARDIO

EXERCISE	DURATION	DISTANCE	CALORIES	HEART RATE

NOTES / NUTRITION

RATING

⚡ BODY STRENGTH	☆☆☆☆☆
🧠 MIND POWER	☆☆☆☆☆

📅 DATE		⏱️ TIME	
⚖️ WEIGHT		📏 BODY FAT	
💪 MUSCLE GROUP		☐ WARM-UP	☐ STRETCH

🏋️ STRENGTH TRAINING

EXERCISE			SET 1	SET 1	SET 1	SET 1	SET 1	SET 1
		REPS						
		WEIGHT						
		REPS						
		WEIGHT						
		REPS						
		WEIGHT						
		REPS						
		WEIGHT						
		REPS						
		WEIGHT						
		REPS						
		WEIGHT						
		REPS						
		WEIGHT						
		REPS						
		WEIGHT						

👟 CARDIO

EXERCISE		DURATION	DISTANCE	CALORIES	HEART RATE

NOTES / NUTRITION	RATING
	⚡ BODY STRENGTH ☆☆☆☆☆
	🧠 MIND POWER ☆☆☆☆☆

📅 DATE		🕐 TIME	
⚖️ WEIGHT		📏 BODY FAT	
💪 MUSCLE GROUP		☐ WARM-UP	☐ STRETCH

🏋️ STRENGTH TRAINING

EXERCISE			SET 1	SET 1	SET 1	SET 1	SET 1	SET 1
		REPS						
		WEIGHT						
		REPS						
		WEIGHT						
		REPS						
		WEIGHT						
		REPS						
		WEIGHT						
		REPS						
		WEIGHT						
		REPS						
		WEIGHT						
		REPS						
		WEIGHT						
		REPS						
		WEIGHT						

👟 CARDIO

EXERCISE	DURATION	DISTANCE	CALORIES	HEART RATE

NOTES / NUTRITION	RATING	
	⚡ BODY STRENGTH	☆☆☆☆☆
	🧠 MIND POWER	☆☆☆☆☆

	DATE			TIME	
	WEIGHT			BODY FAT	
	MUSCLE GROUP		☐ WARM-UP		☐ STRETCH

STRENGTH TRAINING

EXERCISE			SET 1	SET 1	SET 1	SET 1	SET 1	SET 1
		REPS						
		WEIGHT						
		REPS						
		WEIGHT						
		REPS						
		WEIGHT						
		REPS						
		WEIGHT						
		REPS						
		WEIGHT						
		REPS						
		WEIGHT						
		REPS						
		WEIGHT						
		REPS						
		WEIGHT						

CARDIO

EXERCISE		DURATION	DISTANCE	CALORIES	HEART RATE

NOTES / NUTRITION

RATING

BODY STRENGTH	☆☆☆☆☆
MIND POWER	☆☆☆☆☆

📅 DATE		🕐 TIME	
⚖️ WEIGHT		📏 BODY FAT	
💪 MUSCLE GROUP		☐ WARM-UP	☐ STRETCH

🏋️ STRENGTH TRAINING

EXERCISE			SET 1	SET 1	SET 1	SET 1	SET 1	SET 1
		REPS						
		WEIGHT						
		REPS						
		WEIGHT						
		REPS						
		WEIGHT						
		REPS						
		WEIGHT						
		REPS						
		WEIGHT						
		REPS						
		WEIGHT						
		REPS						
		WEIGHT						
		REPS						
		WEIGHT						

👟 CARDIO

EXERCISE	DURATION	DISTANCE	CALORIES	HEART RATE

NOTES / NUTRITION

RATING

⚡	BODY STRENGTH	☆☆☆☆☆
🧠	MIND POWER	☆☆☆☆☆

📅 DATE		⏱️ TIME	
🛁 WEIGHT		📏 BODY FAT	
💪 MUSCLE GROUP		☐ WARM-UP	☐ STRETCH

🏋️ STRENGTH TRAINING

EXERCISE			SET 1	SET 1	SET 1	SET 1	SET 1	SET 1
		REPS						
		WEIGHT						
		REPS						
		WEIGHT						
		REPS						
		WEIGHT						
		REPS						
		WEIGHT						
		REPS						
		WEIGHT						
		REPS						
		WEIGHT						
		REPS						
		WEIGHT						
		REPS						
		WEIGHT						

🏃 CARDIO

EXERCISE		DURATION	DISTANCE	CALORIES	HEART RATE

NOTES / NUTRITION

RATING

⚡ BODY STRENGTH	☆☆☆☆☆
🧠 MIND POWER	☆☆☆☆☆

📅 DATE		⏱️ TIME	
🖼️ WEIGHT		📏 BODY FAT	
💪 MUSCLE GROUP		☐ WARM-UP	☐ STRETCH

🏋️ STRENGTH TRAINING			SET 1	SET 1	SET 1	SET 1	SET 1	SET 1
E X E R C I S E		REPS						
		WEIGHT						
		REPS						
		WEIGHT						
		REPS						
		WEIGHT						
		REPS						
		WEIGHT						
		REPS						
		WEIGHT						
		REPS						
		WEIGHT						
		REPS						
		WEIGHT						
		REPS						
		WEIGHT						

👟 CARDIO		DURATION	DISTANCE	CALORIES	HEART RATE
E X E R C I S E					

NOTES / NUTRITION

RATING	
⚡ BODY STRENGTH	☆☆☆☆☆
🧠 MIND POWER	☆☆☆☆☆

	DATE			TIME	
	WEIGHT			BODY FAT	
	MUSCLE GROUP		☐ WARM-UP		☐ STRETCH

STRENGTH TRAINING

EXERCISE			SET 1	SET 1	SET 1	SET 1	SET 1	SET 1
		REPS						
		WEIGHT						
		REPS						
		WEIGHT						
		REPS						
		WEIGHT						
		REPS						
		WEIGHT						
		REPS						
		WEIGHT						
		REPS						
		WEIGHT						
		REPS						
		WEIGHT						
		REPS						
		WEIGHT						

CARDIO

EXERCISE		DURATION	DISTANCE	CALORIES	HEART RATE

NOTES / NUTRITION

RATING

	BODY STRENGTH	☆☆☆☆☆
	MIND POWER	☆☆☆☆☆

📅 DATE		⏱️ TIME	
⚖️ WEIGHT		📏 BODY FAT	
💪 MUSCLE GROUP		☐ WARM-UP	☐ STRETCH

🏋️ STRENGTH TRAINING

EXERCISE			SET 1	SET 1	SET 1	SET 1	SET 1	SET 1
		REPS						
		WEIGHT						
		REPS						
		WEIGHT						
		REPS						
		WEIGHT						
		REPS						
		WEIGHT						
		REPS						
		WEIGHT						
		REPS						
		WEIGHT						
		REPS						
		WEIGHT						
		REPS						
		WEIGHT						

👟 CARDIO

EXERCISE	DURATION	DISTANCE	CALORIES	HEART RATE

NOTES / NUTRITION

RATING

⚡ BODY STRENGTH	☆☆☆☆☆
🧠 MIND POWER	☆☆☆☆☆

📅 DATE		🕐 TIME	
⚖️ WEIGHT		📏 BODY FAT	
💪 MUSCLE GROUP		☐ WARM-UP	☐ STRETCH

🏋️ STRENGTH TRAINING

EXERCISE			SET 1	SET 1	SET 1	SET 1	SET 1	SET 1
		REPS						
		WEIGHT						
		REPS						
		WEIGHT						
		REPS						
		WEIGHT						
		REPS						
		WEIGHT						
		REPS						
		WEIGHT						
		REPS						
		WEIGHT						
		REPS						
		WEIGHT						
		REPS						
		WEIGHT						

👟 CARDIO

EXERCISE		DURATION	DISTANCE	CALORIES	HEART RATE

NOTES / NUTRITION	RATING
	⚡ BODY STRENGTH ☆☆☆☆☆
	🧠 MIND POWER ☆☆☆☆☆

	DATE		TIME
	WEIGHT		BODY FAT
	MUSCLE GROUP	☐ WARM-UP	☐ STRETCH

STRENGTH TRAINING

EXERCISE			SET 1	SET 1	SET 1	SET 1	SET 1	SET 1
		REPS						
		WEIGHT						
		REPS						
		WEIGHT						
		REPS						
		WEIGHT						
		REPS						
		WEIGHT						
		REPS						
		WEIGHT						
		REPS						
		WEIGHT						
		REPS						
		WEIGHT						
		REPS						
		WEIGHT						

CARDIO

EXERCISE		DURATION	DISTANCE	CALORIES	HEART RATE

NOTES / NUTRITION

RATING

⚡	BODY STRENGTH	☆☆☆☆☆
🧠	MIND POWER	☆☆☆☆☆

	DATE			TIME	
	WEIGHT			BODY FAT	
	MUSCLE GROUP		☐ WARM-UP		☐ STRETCH

STRENGTH TRAINING

EXERCISE			SET 1	SET 1	SET 1	SET 1	SET 1	SET 1
		REPS						
		WEIGHT						
		REPS						
		WEIGHT						
		REPS						
		WEIGHT						
		REPS						
		WEIGHT						
		REPS						
		WEIGHT						
		REPS						
		WEIGHT						
		REPS						
		WEIGHT						
		REPS						
		WEIGHT						

CARDIO

EXERCISE		DURATION	DISTANCE	CALORIES	HEART RATE

NOTES / NUTRITION

RATING

⚡	BODY STRENGTH	☆☆☆☆☆
🧠	MIND POWER	☆☆☆☆☆

📅 DATE		🕚 TIME	
🪑 WEIGHT		📏 BODY FAT	
💪 MUSCLE GROUP		☐ WARM-UP	☐ STRETCH

🏋️ STRENGTH TRAINING

EXERCISE			SET 1	SET 1	SET 1	SET 1	SET 1	SET 1
		REPS						
		WEIGHT						
		REPS						
		WEIGHT						
		REPS						
		WEIGHT						
		REPS						
		WEIGHT						
		REPS						
		WEIGHT						
		REPS						
		WEIGHT						
		REPS						
		WEIGHT						
		REPS						
		WEIGHT						

👟 CARDIO

EXERCISE		DURATION	DISTANCE	CALORIES	HEART RATE

NOTES / NUTRITION	RATING
	⚡ BODY STRENGTH ☆☆☆☆☆
	🧠 MIND POWER ☆☆☆☆☆

📅 DATE		⏱ TIME	
⬜ WEIGHT		📏 BODY FAT	
💪 MUSCLE GROUP		☐ WARM-UP	☐ STRETCH

🏋 STRENGTH TRAINING

EXERCISE			SET 1	SET 1	SET 1	SET 1	SET 1	SET 1
		REPS						
		WEIGHT						
		REPS						
		WEIGHT						
		REPS						
		WEIGHT						
		REPS						
		WEIGHT						
		REPS						
		WEIGHT						
		REPS						
		WEIGHT						
		REPS						
		WEIGHT						
		REPS						
		WEIGHT						

👟 CARDIO

EXERCISE	DURATION	DISTANCE	CALORIES	HEART RATE

NOTES / NUTRITION

RATING

⚡ BODY STRENGTH	☆☆☆☆☆
🧠 MIND POWER	☆☆☆☆☆

📅 DATE		⏱️ TIME	
🖼️ WEIGHT		🧵 BODY FAT	
💪 MUSCLE GROUP		☐ WARM-UP	☐ STRETCH

🏋️ STRENGTH TRAINING

EXERCISE			SET 1	SET 1	SET 1	SET 1	SET 1	SET 1
		REPS						
		WEIGHT						
		REPS						
		WEIGHT						
		REPS						
		WEIGHT						
		REPS						
		WEIGHT						
		REPS						
		WEIGHT						
		REPS						
		WEIGHT						
		REPS						
		WEIGHT						
		REPS						
		WEIGHT						

👟 CARDIO

EXERCISE	DURATION	DISTANCE	CALORIES	HEART RATE

NOTES / NUTRITION

RATING

⚡ BODY STRENGTH	☆☆☆☆☆
🧠 MIND POWER	☆☆☆☆☆

📅 DATE		⏱️ TIME	
⚖️ WEIGHT		📏 BODY FAT	
💪 MUSCLE GROUP		☐ WARM-UP	☐ STRETCH

🏋️ STRENGTH TRAINING

EXERCISE			SET 1	SET 1	SET 1	SET 1	SET 1	SET 1
		REPS						
		WEIGHT						
		REPS						
		WEIGHT						
		REPS						
		WEIGHT						
		REPS						
		WEIGHT						
		REPS						
		WEIGHT						
		REPS						
		WEIGHT						
		REPS						
		WEIGHT						
		REPS						
		WEIGHT						

👟 CARDIO

EXERCISE		DURATION	DISTANCE	CALORIES	HEART RATE

NOTES / NUTRITION	RATING
	⚡ BODY STRENGTH ☆☆☆☆☆
	🧠 MIND POWER ☆☆☆☆☆

📅 DATE		⏱️ TIME	
⚖️ WEIGHT		📏 BODY FAT	
💪 MUSCLE GROUP		☐ WARM-UP	☐ STRETCH

🏋️ STRENGTH TRAINING

EXERCISE			SET 1	SET 1	SET 1	SET 1	SET 1	SET 1
		REPS						
		WEIGHT						
		REPS						
		WEIGHT						
		REPS						
		WEIGHT						
		REPS						
		WEIGHT						
		REPS						
		WEIGHT						
		REPS						
		WEIGHT						
		REPS						
		WEIGHT						
		REPS						
		WEIGHT						

👟 CARDIO

EXERCISE	DURATION	DISTANCE	CALORIES	HEART RATE

NOTES / NUTRITION	RATING	
	⚡ BODY STRENGTH	☆☆☆☆☆
	🧠 MIND POWER	☆☆☆☆☆

	DATE			TIME	
	WEIGHT			BODY FAT	
	MUSCLE GROUP		☐ WARM-UP		☐ STRETCH

STRENGTH TRAINING

EXERCISE			SET 1	SET 1	SET 1	SET 1	SET 1	SET 1
		REPS						
		WEIGHT						
		REPS						
		WEIGHT						
		REPS						
		WEIGHT						
		REPS						
		WEIGHT						
		REPS						
		WEIGHT						
		REPS						
		WEIGHT						
		REPS						
		WEIGHT						
		REPS						
		WEIGHT						

CARDIO

EXERCISE		DURATION	DISTANCE	CALORIES	HEART RATE

NOTES / NUTRITION

RATING

	BODY STRENGTH	☆☆☆☆☆
	MIND POWER	☆☆☆☆☆

📅 DATE		🕙 TIME	
🖼 WEIGHT		📏 BODY FAT	
💪 MUSCLE GROUP		☐ WARM-UP	☐ STRETCH

🏋 STRENGTH TRAINING

EXERCISE			SET 1	SET 1	SET 1	SET 1	SET 1	SET 1
		REPS						
		WEIGHT						
		REPS						
		WEIGHT						
		REPS						
		WEIGHT						
		REPS						
		WEIGHT						
		REPS						
		WEIGHT						
		REPS						
		WEIGHT						
		REPS						
		WEIGHT						
		REPS						
		WEIGHT						

👟 CARDIO

EXERCISE		DURATION	DISTANCE	CALORIES	HEART RATE

NOTES / NUTRITION	RATING	
	⚡ BODY STRENGTH	☆☆☆☆☆
	🧠 MIND POWER	☆☆☆☆☆

📅 DATE		⏱️ TIME	
⚖️ WEIGHT		📏 BODY FAT	
💪 MUSCLE GROUP		☐ WARM-UP	☐ STRETCH

🏋️ STRENGTH TRAINING

EXERCISE			SET 1	SET 1	SET 1	SET 1	SET 1	SET 1
		REPS						
		WEIGHT						
		REPS						
		WEIGHT						
		REPS						
		WEIGHT						
		REPS						
		WEIGHT						
		REPS						
		WEIGHT						
		REPS						
		WEIGHT						
		REPS						
		WEIGHT						
		REPS						
		WEIGHT						

👟 CARDIO

EXERCISE		DURATION	DISTANCE	CALORIES	HEART RATE

NOTES / NUTRITION	RATING	
	⚡ BODY STRENGTH	☆☆☆☆☆
	🧠 MIND POWER	☆☆☆☆☆

	DATE			TIME
	WEIGHT			BODY FAT
	MUSCLE GROUP		☐ WARM-UP	☐ STRETCH

STRENGTH TRAINING

EXERCISE			SET 1	SET 1	SET 1	SET 1	SET 1	SET 1
		REPS						
		WEIGHT						
		REPS						
		WEIGHT						
		REPS						
		WEIGHT						
		REPS						
		WEIGHT						
		REPS						
		WEIGHT						
		REPS						
		WEIGHT						
		REPS						
		WEIGHT						
		REPS						
		WEIGHT						

CARDIO

EXERCISE		DURATION	DISTANCE	CALORIES	HEART RATE

NOTES / NUTRITION

RATING

	BODY STRENGTH	☆☆☆☆☆
	MIND POWER	☆☆☆☆☆

📅 DATE	🕐 TIME
🪣 WEIGHT	📏 BODY FAT
💪 MUSCLE GROUP	☐ WARM-UP ☐ STRETCH

🏋 STRENGTH TRAINING

EXERCISE			SET 1	SET 1	SET 1	SET 1	SET 1	SET 1
		REPS						
		WEIGHT						
		REPS						
		WEIGHT						
		REPS						
		WEIGHT						
		REPS						
		WEIGHT						
		REPS						
		WEIGHT						
		REPS						
		WEIGHT						
		REPS						
		WEIGHT						
		REPS						
		WEIGHT						

👟 CARDIO

EXERCISE	DURATION	DISTANCE	CALORIES	HEART RATE

NOTES / NUTRITION

RATING

⚡ BODY STRENGTH	☆☆☆☆☆
🧠 MIND POWER	☆☆☆☆☆

	DATE			TIME
	WEIGHT			BODY FAT
	MUSCLE GROUP		☐ WARM-UP	☐ STRETCH

STRENGTH TRAINING

EXERCISE			SET 1	SET 1	SET 1	SET 1	SET 1	SET 1
		REPS						
		WEIGHT						
		REPS						
		WEIGHT						
		REPS						
		WEIGHT						
		REPS						
		WEIGHT						
		REPS						
		WEIGHT						
		REPS						
		WEIGHT						
		REPS						
		WEIGHT						
		REPS						
		WEIGHT						

CARDIO

EXERCISE		DURATION	DISTANCE	CALORIES	HEART RATE

NOTES / NUTRITION	RATING
	BODY STRENGTH ☆☆☆☆☆
	MIND POWER ☆☆☆☆☆

	DATE		TIME
	WEIGHT		BODY FAT
	MUSCLE GROUP	☐ WARM-UP	☐ STRETCH

STRENGTH TRAINING

EXERCISE			SET 1	SET 1	SET 1	SET 1	SET 1	SET 1
		REPS						
		WEIGHT						
		REPS						
		WEIGHT						
		REPS						
		WEIGHT						
		REPS						
		WEIGHT						
		REPS						
		WEIGHT						
		REPS						
		WEIGHT						
		REPS						
		WEIGHT						
		REPS						
		WEIGHT						

CARDIO

EXERCISE		DURATION	DISTANCE	CALORIES	HEART RATE

NOTES / NUTRITION

RATING

	BODY STRENGTH	☆☆☆☆☆
	MIND POWER	☆☆☆☆☆

📅 DATE		🕐 TIME	
⚖️ WEIGHT		📏 BODY FAT	
💪 MUSCLE GROUP		☐ WARM-UP	☐ STRETCH

🏋️ STRENGTH TRAINING

EXERCISE			SET 1	SET 1	SET 1	SET 1	SET 1	SET 1
		REPS						
		WEIGHT						
		REPS						
		WEIGHT						
		REPS						
		WEIGHT						
		REPS						
		WEIGHT						
		REPS						
		WEIGHT						
		REPS						
		WEIGHT						
		REPS						
		WEIGHT						
		REPS						
		WEIGHT						

👟 CARDIO

EXERCISE	DURATION	DISTANCE	CALORIES	HEART RATE

NOTES / NUTRITION	RATING	
	⚡ BODY STRENGTH	☆☆☆☆☆
	🧠 MIND POWER	☆☆☆☆☆

	DATE			TIME	
	WEIGHT			BODY FAT	
	MUSCLE GROUP		☐ WARM-UP		☐ STRETCH

STRENGTH TRAINING

EXERCISE			SET 1	SET 1	SET 1	SET 1	SET 1	SET 1
		REPS						
		WEIGHT						
		REPS						
		WEIGHT						
		REPS						
		WEIGHT						
		REPS						
		WEIGHT						
		REPS						
		WEIGHT						
		REPS						
		WEIGHT						
		REPS						
		WEIGHT						
		REPS						
		WEIGHT						

CARDIO

EXERCISE		DURATION	DISTANCE	CALORIES	HEART RATE

NOTES / NUTRITION

RATING

	BODY STRENGTH	☆☆☆☆☆
	MIND POWER	☆☆☆☆☆

📅 DATE		⏱️ TIME	
🔲 WEIGHT		📏 BODY FAT	
💪 MUSCLE GROUP		☐ WARM-UP	☐ STRETCH

🏋️ STRENGTH TRAINING			SET 1	SET 1	SET 1	SET 1	SET 1	SET 1
EXERCISE		REPS						
		WEIGHT						
		REPS						
		WEIGHT						
		REPS						
		WEIGHT						
		REPS						
		WEIGHT						
		REPS						
		WEIGHT						
		REPS						
		WEIGHT						
		REPS						
		WEIGHT						
		REPS						
		WEIGHT						

👟 CARDIO		DURATION	DISTANCE	CALORIES	HEART RATE
EXERCISE					

NOTES / NUTRITION

RATING	
⚡ BODY STRENGTH	☆☆☆☆☆
🧠 MIND POWER	☆☆☆☆☆

📅 DATE		⏱ TIME	
⚖ WEIGHT		📏 BODY FAT	
💪 MUSCLE GROUP		☐ WARM-UP	☐ STRETCH

🏋 STRENGTH TRAINING

EXERCISE			SET 1	SET 1	SET 1	SET 1	SET 1	SET 1
		REPS						
		WEIGHT						
		REPS						
		WEIGHT						
		REPS						
		WEIGHT						
		REPS						
		WEIGHT						
		REPS						
		WEIGHT						
		REPS						
		WEIGHT						
		REPS						
		WEIGHT						
		REPS						
		WEIGHT						

👟 CARDIO

EXERCISE		DURATION	DISTANCE	CALORIES	HEART RATE

NOTES / NUTRITION	RATING	
	⚡ BODY STRENGTH	☆☆☆☆☆
	🧠 MIND POWER	☆☆☆☆☆

📅 DATE		⏱️ TIME	
⚖️ WEIGHT		📏 BODY FAT	
💪 MUSCLE GROUP		☐ WARM-UP	☐ STRETCH

🏋️ STRENGTH TRAINING

EXERCISE			SET 1	SET 1	SET 1	SET 1	SET 1	SET 1
		REPS						
		WEIGHT						
		REPS						
		WEIGHT						
		REPS						
		WEIGHT						
		REPS						
		WEIGHT						
		REPS						
		WEIGHT						
		REPS						
		WEIGHT						
		REPS						
		WEIGHT						
		REPS						
		WEIGHT						

👟 CARDIO

EXERCISE	DURATION	DISTANCE	CALORIES	HEART RATE

NOTES / NUTRITION

RATING	
⚡ BODY STRENGTH	☆☆☆☆☆
🧠 MIND POWER	☆☆☆☆☆

📅 DATE		⏱ TIME	
⚖ WEIGHT		📏 BODY FAT	
💪 MUSCLE GROUP		☐ WARM-UP	☐ STRETCH

🏋 STRENGTH TRAINING

EXERCISE			SET 1	SET 1	SET 1	SET 1	SET 1	SET 1
		REPS						
		WEIGHT						
		REPS						
		WEIGHT						
		REPS						
		WEIGHT						
		REPS						
		WEIGHT						
		REPS						
		WEIGHT						
		REPS						
		WEIGHT						
		REPS						
		WEIGHT						
		REPS						
		WEIGHT						

👟 CARDIO

EXERCISE		DURATION	DISTANCE	CALORIES	HEART RATE

NOTES / NUTRITION

RATING

⚡ BODY STRENGTH	☆☆☆☆☆
🧠 MIND POWER	☆☆☆☆☆

	DATE		TIME
	WEIGHT		BODY FAT
	MUSCLE GROUP	☐ WARM-UP	☐ STRETCH

🏋 STRENGTH TRAINING

EXERCISE			SET 1	SET 1	SET 1	SET 1	SET 1	SET 1
		REPS						
		WEIGHT						
		REPS						
		WEIGHT						
		REPS						
		WEIGHT						
		REPS						
		WEIGHT						
		REPS						
		WEIGHT						
		REPS						
		WEIGHT						
		REPS						
		WEIGHT						
		REPS						
		WEIGHT						

👟 CARDIO

EXERCISE		DURATION	DISTANCE	CALORIES	HEART RATE

NOTES / NUTRITION

RATING

⚡	BODY STRENGTH	☆☆☆☆☆
🧠	MIND POWER	☆☆☆☆☆

📅 DATE		⏱️ TIME	
⚖️ WEIGHT		📏 BODY FAT	
💪 MUSCLE GROUP		☐ WARM-UP	☐ STRETCH

🏋️ STRENGTH TRAINING

EXERCISE			SET 1	SET 1	SET 1	SET 1	SET 1	SET 1
		REPS						
		WEIGHT						
		REPS						
		WEIGHT						
		REPS						
		WEIGHT						
		REPS						
		WEIGHT						
		REPS						
		WEIGHT						
		REPS						
		WEIGHT						
		REPS						
		WEIGHT						
		REPS						
		WEIGHT						

👟 CARDIO

EXERCISE		DURATION	DISTANCE	CALORIES	HEART RATE

NOTES / NUTRITION	RATING	
	⚡ BODY STRENGTH	☆☆☆☆☆
	🧠 MIND POWER	☆☆☆☆☆

📅 DATE		⏱ TIME	
⬜ WEIGHT		📏 BODY FAT	
💪 MUSCLE GROUP		☐ WARM-UP	☐ STRETCH

🏋 STRENGTH TRAINING

EXERCISE			SET 1	SET 1	SET 1	SET 1	SET 1	SET 1
		REPS						
		WEIGHT						
		REPS						
		WEIGHT						
		REPS						
		WEIGHT						
		REPS						
		WEIGHT						
		REPS						
		WEIGHT						
		REPS						
		WEIGHT						
		REPS						
		WEIGHT						
		REPS						
		WEIGHT						

👟 CARDIO

EXERCISE	DURATION	DISTANCE	CALORIES	HEART RATE

NOTES / NUTRITION

RATING

⚡ BODY STRENGTH	☆☆☆☆☆
🧠 MIND POWER	☆☆☆☆☆

	DATE			TIME	
	WEIGHT			BODY FAT	
	MUSCLE GROUP		☐ WARM-UP		☐ STRETCH

STRENGTH TRAINING

EXERCISE			SET 1	SET 1	SET 1	SET 1	SET 1	SET 1
		REPS						
		WEIGHT						
		REPS						
		WEIGHT						
		REPS						
		WEIGHT						
		REPS						
		WEIGHT						
		REPS						
		WEIGHT						
		REPS						
		WEIGHT						
		REPS						
		WEIGHT						
		REPS						
		WEIGHT						

CARDIO

EXERCISE		DURATION	DISTANCE	CALORIES	HEART RATE

NOTES / NUTRITION	RATING	
	BODY STRENGTH	☆☆☆☆☆
	MIND POWER	☆☆☆☆☆

📅 DATE		⏱ TIME	
⚖ WEIGHT		🩹 BODY FAT	
💪 MUSCLE GROUP		☐ WARM-UP	☐ STRETCH

🏋 STRENGTH TRAINING			SET 1	SET 1	SET 1	SET 1	SET 1	SET 1
EXERCISE		REPS						
		WEIGHT						
		REPS						
		WEIGHT						
		REPS						
		WEIGHT						
		REPS						
		WEIGHT						
		REPS						
		WEIGHT						
		REPS						
		WEIGHT						
		REPS						
		WEIGHT						
		REPS						
		WEIGHT						

👟 CARDIO		DURATION	DISTANCE	CALORIES	HEART RATE
EXERCISE					

NOTES / NUTRITION

RATING	
⚡ BODY STRENGTH	☆☆☆☆☆
🧠 MIND POWER	☆☆☆☆☆

📅 DATE		🕐 TIME	
⚖️ WEIGHT		📏 BODY FAT	
💪 MUSCLE GROUP		☐ WARM-UP	☐ STRETCH

🏋️ STRENGTH TRAINING

EXERCISE			SET 1	SET 1	SET 1	SET 1	SET 1	SET 1
		REPS						
		WEIGHT						
		REPS						
		WEIGHT						
		REPS						
		WEIGHT						
		REPS						
		WEIGHT						
		REPS						
		WEIGHT						
		REPS						
		WEIGHT						
		REPS						
		WEIGHT						
		REPS						
		WEIGHT						

👟 CARDIO

EXERCISE	DURATION	DISTANCE	CALORIES	HEART RATE

NOTES / NUTRITION

RATING

⚡	BODY STRENGTH	☆☆☆☆☆
🧠	MIND POWER	☆☆☆☆☆

📅 DATE		⏱️ TIME	
⚖️ WEIGHT		📏 BODY FAT	
💪 MUSCLE GROUP		☐ WARM-UP	☐ STRETCH

🏋️ STRENGTH TRAINING

EXERCISE			SET 1	SET 1	SET 1	SET 1	SET 1	SET 1
		REPS						
		WEIGHT						
		REPS						
		WEIGHT						
		REPS						
		WEIGHT						
		REPS						
		WEIGHT						
		REPS						
		WEIGHT						
		REPS						
		WEIGHT						
		REPS						
		WEIGHT						
		REPS						
		WEIGHT						

👟 CARDIO

EXERCISE		DURATION	DISTANCE	CALORIES	HEART RATE

NOTES / NUTRITION

RATING

⚡ BODY STRENGTH	☆☆☆☆☆
🧠 MIND POWER	☆☆☆☆☆

📅 DATE		⏱ TIME	
⚖ WEIGHT		📏 BODY FAT	
💪 MUSCLE GROUP		☐ WARM-UP	☐ STRETCH

🏋 STRENGTH TRAINING

			SET 1	SET 1	SET 1	SET 1	SET 1	SET 1
EXERCISE		REPS						
		WEIGHT						
		REPS						
		WEIGHT						
		REPS						
		WEIGHT						
		REPS						
		WEIGHT						
		REPS						
		WEIGHT						
		REPS						
		WEIGHT						
		REPS						
		WEIGHT						
		REPS						
		WEIGHT						

👟 CARDIO

		DURATION	DISTANCE	CALORIES	HEART RATE
EXERCISE					

NOTES / NUTRITION

RATING	
⚡ BODY STRENGTH	☆☆☆☆☆
🧠 MIND POWER	☆☆☆☆☆

📅 DATE		⏱ TIME	
⚖ WEIGHT		📏 BODY FAT	
💪 MUSCLE GROUP		☐ WARM-UP	☐ STRETCH

🏋 STRENGTH TRAINING

EXERCISE			SET 1	SET 1	SET 1	SET 1	SET 1	SET 1
		REPS						
		WEIGHT						
		REPS						
		WEIGHT						
		REPS						
		WEIGHT						
		REPS						
		WEIGHT						
		REPS						
		WEIGHT						
		REPS						
		WEIGHT						
		REPS						
		WEIGHT						
		REPS						
		WEIGHT						

👟 CARDIO

EXERCISE		DURATION	DISTANCE	CALORIES	HEART RATE

NOTES / NUTRITION	RATING
	⚡ BODY STRENGTH ☆☆☆☆☆
	🧠 MIND POWER ☆☆☆☆☆

📅 DATE		⏱️ TIME	
⚖️ WEIGHT		📏 BODY FAT	
💪 MUSCLE GROUP		☐ WARM-UP	☐ STRETCH

🏋️ STRENGTH TRAINING			SET 1	SET 1	SET 1	SET 1	SET 1	SET 1
E X E R C I S E		REPS						
		WEIGHT						
		REPS						
		WEIGHT						
		REPS						
		WEIGHT						
		REPS						
		WEIGHT						
		REPS						
		WEIGHT						
		REPS						
		WEIGHT						
		REPS						
		WEIGHT						
		REPS						
		WEIGHT						

👟 CARDIO		DURATION	DISTANCE	CALORIES	HEART RATE
E X E R C I S E					

NOTES / NUTRITION

RATING	
⚡ BODY STRENGTH	☆☆☆☆☆
🧠 MIND POWER	☆☆☆☆☆

📅 DATE		🕐 TIME	
⚖️ WEIGHT		📏 BODY FAT	
💪 MUSCLE GROUP		☐ WARM-UP	☐ STRETCH

🏋️ STRENGTH TRAINING			SET 1	SET 1	SET 1	SET 1	SET 1	SET 1
EXERCISE		REPS						
		WEIGHT						
		REPS						
		WEIGHT						
		REPS						
		WEIGHT						
		REPS						
		WEIGHT						
		REPS						
		WEIGHT						
		REPS						
		WEIGHT						
		REPS						
		WEIGHT						
		REPS						
		WEIGHT						

👟 CARDIO	DURATION	DISTANCE	CALORIES	HEART RATE
EXERCISE				

NOTES / NUTRITION

RATING	
⚡ BODY STRENGTH	☆☆☆☆☆
🧠 MIND POWER	☆☆☆☆☆

📅 DATE		⏱️ TIME	
⚖️ WEIGHT		📏 BODY FAT	
💪 MUSCLE GROUP		☐ WARM-UP	☐ STRETCH

🏋️ STRENGTH TRAINING

EXERCISE			SET 1	SET 1	SET 1	SET 1	SET 1	SET 1
		REPS						
		WEIGHT						
		REPS						
		WEIGHT						
		REPS						
		WEIGHT						
		REPS						
		WEIGHT						
		REPS						
		WEIGHT						
		REPS						
		WEIGHT						
		REPS						
		WEIGHT						
		REPS						
		WEIGHT						

👟 CARDIO

EXERCISE		DURATION	DISTANCE	CALORIES	HEART RATE

NOTES / NUTRITION

RATING	
⚡ BODY STRENGTH	☆☆☆☆☆
🧠 MIND POWER	☆☆☆☆☆

📅 DATE		⏱️ TIME	
⚖️ WEIGHT		📏 BODY FAT	
💪 MUSCLE GROUP		☐ WARM-UP	☐ STRETCH

🏋️ STRENGTH TRAINING

EXERCISE			SET 1	SET 1	SET 1	SET 1	SET 1	SET 1
		REPS						
		WEIGHT						
		REPS						
		WEIGHT						
		REPS						
		WEIGHT						
		REPS						
		WEIGHT						
		REPS						
		WEIGHT						
		REPS						
		WEIGHT						
		REPS						
		WEIGHT						
		REPS						
		WEIGHT						

👟 CARDIO

EXERCISE	DURATION	DISTANCE	CALORIES	HEART RATE

NOTES / NUTRITION	RATING	
	⚡ BODY STRENGTH	☆☆☆☆☆
	🧠 MIND POWER	☆☆☆☆☆

	DATE		TIME
	WEIGHT		BODY FAT
	MUSCLE GROUP	☐ WARM-UP	☐ STRETCH

STRENGTH TRAINING

EXERCISE			SET 1	SET 1	SET 1	SET 1	SET 1	SET 1
		REPS						
		WEIGHT						
		REPS						
		WEIGHT						
		REPS						
		WEIGHT						
		REPS						
		WEIGHT						
		REPS						
		WEIGHT						
		REPS						
		WEIGHT						
		REPS						
		WEIGHT						
		REPS						
		WEIGHT						

CARDIO

EXERCISE		DURATION	DISTANCE	CALORIES	HEART RATE

NOTES / NUTRITION	RATING
	⚡ BODY STRENGTH ☆☆☆☆☆
	🧠 MIND POWER ☆☆☆☆☆

	DATE			TIME	
	WEIGHT			BODY FAT	
	MUSCLE GROUP		☐ WARM-UP	☐ STRETCH	

STRENGTH TRAINING

EXERCISE			SET 1	SET 1	SET 1	SET 1	SET 1	SET 1
		REPS						
		WEIGHT						
		REPS						
		WEIGHT						
		REPS						
		WEIGHT						
		REPS						
		WEIGHT						
		REPS						
		WEIGHT						
		REPS						
		WEIGHT						
		REPS						
		WEIGHT						
		REPS						
		WEIGHT						

CARDIO

EXERCISE	DURATION	DISTANCE	CALORIES	HEART RATE

NOTES / NUTRITION

RATING

	BODY STRENGTH	☆☆☆☆☆
	MIND POWER	☆☆☆☆☆

📅 DATE		⏱️ TIME	
🪑 WEIGHT		📏 BODY FAT	
💪 MUSCLE GROUP		☐ WARM-UP	☐ STRETCH

🏋️ STRENGTH TRAINING

EXERCISE			SET 1	SET 1	SET 1	SET 1	SET 1	SET 1
		REPS						
		WEIGHT						
		REPS						
		WEIGHT						
		REPS						
		WEIGHT						
		REPS						
		WEIGHT						
		REPS						
		WEIGHT						
		REPS						
		WEIGHT						
		REPS						
		WEIGHT						
		REPS						
		WEIGHT						

👟 CARDIO

EXERCISE		DURATION	DISTANCE	CALORIES	HEART RATE

NOTES / NUTRITION	RATING
	⚡ BODY STRENGTH ☆☆☆☆☆
	🧠 MIND POWER ☆☆☆☆☆

📅 DATE		🕑 TIME	
⚖️ WEIGHT		📏 BODY FAT	
💪 MUSCLE GROUP		☐ WARM-UP	☐ STRETCH

🏋️ STRENGTH TRAINING

EXERCISE			SET 1	SET 1	SET 1	SET 1	SET 1	SET 1
		REPS						
		WEIGHT						
		REPS						
		WEIGHT						
		REPS						
		WEIGHT						
		REPS						
		WEIGHT						
		REPS						
		WEIGHT						
		REPS						
		WEIGHT						
		REPS						
		WEIGHT						
		REPS						
		WEIGHT						

👟 CARDIO

EXERCISE	DURATION	DISTANCE	CALORIES	HEART RATE

NOTES / NUTRITION

RATING

⚡ BODY STRENGTH	☆☆☆☆☆
🧠 MIND POWER	☆☆☆☆☆

📅 DATE		⏱ TIME	
⚖ WEIGHT		📏 BODY FAT	
💪 MUSCLE GROUP		☐ WARM-UP	☐ STRETCH

🏋 STRENGTH TRAINING

EXERCISE			SET 1	SET 1	SET 1	SET 1	SET 1	SET 1
		REPS						
		WEIGHT						
		REPS						
		WEIGHT						
		REPS						
		WEIGHT						
		REPS						
		WEIGHT						
		REPS						
		WEIGHT						
		REPS						
		WEIGHT						
		REPS						
		WEIGHT						
		REPS						
		WEIGHT						

👟 CARDIO

EXERCISE		DURATION	DISTANCE	CALORIES	HEART RATE

NOTES / NUTRITION	RATING	
	⚡ BODY STRENGTH	☆☆☆☆☆
	🧠 MIND POWER	☆☆☆☆☆

📅 DATE		🕐 TIME	
⚖️ WEIGHT		📏 BODY FAT	
💪 MUSCLE GROUP		☐ WARM-UP	☐ STRETCH

🏋️ STRENGTH TRAINING

EXERCISE			SET 1	SET 1	SET 1	SET 1	SET 1	SET 1
		REPS						
		WEIGHT						
		REPS						
		WEIGHT						
		REPS						
		WEIGHT						
		REPS						
		WEIGHT						
		REPS						
		WEIGHT						
		REPS						
		WEIGHT						
		REPS						
		WEIGHT						
		REPS						
		WEIGHT						

👟 CARDIO

EXERCISE		DURATION	DISTANCE	CALORIES	HEART RATE

NOTES / NUTRITION		RATING	
		⚡ BODY STRENGTH	☆☆☆☆☆
		🧠 MIND POWER	☆☆☆☆☆

📅 DATE		⏱ TIME	
🖼 WEIGHT		📏 BODY FAT	
💪 MUSCLE GROUP		☐ WARM-UP	☐ STRETCH

🏋 STRENGTH TRAINING

EXERCISE			SET 1	SET 1	SET 1	SET 1	SET 1	SET 1
		REPS						
		WEIGHT						
		REPS						
		WEIGHT						
		REPS						
		WEIGHT						
		REPS						
		WEIGHT						
		REPS						
		WEIGHT						
		REPS						
		WEIGHT						
		REPS						
		WEIGHT						
		REPS						
		WEIGHT						

👟 CARDIO

EXERCISE		DURATION	DISTANCE	CALORIES	HEART RATE

NOTES / NUTRITION

RATING

⚡ BODY STRENGTH	☆☆☆☆☆
🧠 MIND POWER	☆☆☆☆☆

📅 DATE		⏱ TIME	
⬜ WEIGHT		📏 BODY FAT	
💪 MUSCLE GROUP		☐ WARM-UP	☐ STRETCH

🏋 STRENGTH TRADING

EXERCISE			SET 1	SET 1	SET 1	SET 1	SET 1	SET 1
		REPS						
		WEIGHT						
		REPS						
		WEIGHT						
		REPS						
		WEIGHT						
		REPS						
		WEIGHT						
		REPS						
		WEIGHT						
		REPS						
		WEIGHT						
		REPS						
		WEIGHT						
		REPS						
		WEIGHT						

👟 CARDIO

EXERCISE	DURATION	DISTANCE	CALORIES	HEART RATE

NOTES / NUTRITION

RATING

⚡ BODY STRENGTH	☆☆☆☆☆
🧠 MIND POWER	☆☆☆☆☆

📅 DATE		🕐 TIME	
⚖ WEIGHT		📏 BODY FAT	
💪 MUSCLE GROUP		☐ WARM-UP	☐ STRETCH

🏋 STRENGTH TRAINING			SET 1	SET 1	SET 1	SET 1	SET 1	SET 1
EXERCISE		REPS						
		WEIGHT						
		REPS						
		WEIGHT						
		REPS						
		WEIGHT						
		REPS						
		WEIGHT						
		REPS						
		WEIGHT						
		REPS						
		WEIGHT						
		REPS						
		WEIGHT						
		REPS						
		WEIGHT						

👟 CARDIO		DURATION	DISTANCE	CALORIES	HEART RATE
EXERCISE					

NOTES / NUTRITION

RATING	
⚡ BODY STRENGTH	☆☆☆☆☆
🧠 MIND POWER	☆☆☆☆☆

📅 DATE		⏱️ TIME
⚖️ WEIGHT		📏 BODY FAT
💪 MUSCLE GROUP		☐ WARM-UP ☐ STRETCH

🏋️ STRENGTH TRAINING

EXERCISE			SET 1	SET 1	SET 1	SET 1	SET 1	SET 1
		REPS						
		WEIGHT						
		REPS						
		WEIGHT						
		REPS						
		WEIGHT						
		REPS						
		WEIGHT						
		REPS						
		WEIGHT						
		REPS						
		WEIGHT						
		REPS						
		WEIGHT						
		REPS						
		WEIGHT						

👟 CARDIO

EXERCISE	DURATION	DISTANCE	CALORIES	HEART RATE

NOTES / NUTRITION	RATING	
	⚡ BODY STRENGTH	☆☆☆☆☆
	🧠 MIND POWER	☆☆☆☆☆

📅 DATE		⏱️ TIME	
⚖️ WEIGHT		📏 BODY FAT	
💪 MUSCLE GROUP		☐ WARM-UP	☐ STRETCH

🏋️ STRENGTH TRAINING

EXERCISE			SET 1	SET 1	SET 1	SET 1	SET 1	SET 1
		REPS						
		WEIGHT						
		REPS						
		WEIGHT						
		REPS						
		WEIGHT						
		REPS						
		WEIGHT						
		REPS						
		WEIGHT						
		REPS						
		WEIGHT						
		REPS						
		WEIGHT						
		REPS						
		WEIGHT						

👟 CARDIO

EXERCISE		DURATION	DISTANCE	CALORIES	HEART RATE

NOTES / NUTRITION

RATING

⚡	BODY STRENGTH	☆☆☆☆☆
🧠	MIND POWER	☆☆☆☆☆

	DATE			TIME	
	WEIGHT			BODY FAT	
	MUSCLE GROUP		☐ WARM-UP		☐ STRETCH

STRENGTH TRAINING

EXERCISE			SET 1	SET 1	SET 1	SET 1	SET 1	SET 1
		REPS						
		WEIGHT						
		REPS						
		WEIGHT						
		REPS						
		WEIGHT						
		REPS						
		WEIGHT						
		REPS						
		WEIGHT						
		REPS						
		WEIGHT						
		REPS						
		WEIGHT						
		REPS						
		WEIGHT						

CARDIO

EXERCISE		DURATION	DISTANCE	CALORIES	HEART RATE

NOTES / NUTRITION

RATING

	BODY STRENGTH	☆☆☆☆☆
	MIND POWER	☆☆☆☆☆

📅 DATE		⏱️ TIME	
⚖️ WEIGHT		📏 BODY FAT	
💪 MUSCLE GROUP		☐ WARM-UP	☐ STRETCH

🏋️ STRENGTH TRAINING

EXERCISE			SET 1	SET 1	SET 1	SET 1	SET 1	SET 1
		REPS						
		WEIGHT						
		REPS						
		WEIGHT						
		REPS						
		WEIGHT						
		REPS						
		WEIGHT						
		REPS						
		WEIGHT						
		REPS						
		WEIGHT						
		REPS						
		WEIGHT						
		REPS						
		WEIGHT						

👟 CARDIO

EXERCISE		DURATION	DISTANCE	CALORIES	HEART RATE

NOTES / NUTRITION	RATING	
	⚡ BODY STRENGTH	☆☆☆☆☆
	🧠 MIND POWER	☆☆☆☆☆

📅 DATE		🕗 TIME	
🖼 WEIGHT		📏 BODY FAT	
💪 MUSCLE GROUP		☐ WARM-UP	☐ STRETCH

🏋 STRENGTH TRAINING			SET 1	SET 1	SET 1	SET 1	SET 1	SET 1
EXERCISE		REPS						
		WEIGHT						
		REPS						
		WEIGHT						
		REPS						
		WEIGHT						
		REPS						
		WEIGHT						
		REPS						
		WEIGHT						
		REPS						
		WEIGHT						
		REPS						
		WEIGHT						
		REPS						
		WEIGHT						

👟 CARDIO	DURATION	DISTANCE	CALORIES	HEART RATE
EXERCISE				

NOTES / NUTRITION

RATING	
⚡ BODY STRENGTH	☆☆☆☆☆
🧠 MIND POWER	☆☆☆☆☆

📅 DATE		⏱️ TIME	
⚖️ WEIGHT		📏 BODY FAT	
💪 MUSCLE GROUP		☐ WARM-UP	☐ STRETCH

🏋️ STRENGTH TRAINING

			SET 1	SET 1	SET 1	SET 1	SET 1	SET 1
EXERCISE		REPS						
		WEIGHT						
		REPS						
		WEIGHT						
		REPS						
		WEIGHT						
		REPS						
		WEIGHT						
		REPS						
		WEIGHT						
		REPS						
		WEIGHT						
		REPS						
		WEIGHT						
		REPS						
		WEIGHT						

👟 CARDIO

		DURATION	DISTANCE	CALORIES	HEART RATE
EXERCISE					

NOTES / NUTRITION

RATING

⚡	BODY STRENGTH	☆☆☆☆☆
🧠	MIND POWER	☆☆☆☆☆

📅 DATE		⏱️ TIME	
⚖️ WEIGHT		📏 BODY FAT	
💪 MUSCLE GROUP		☐ WARM-UP	☐ STRETCH

🏋️ STRENGTH TRAINING

EXERCISE			SET 1	SET 1	SET 1	SET 1	SET 1	SET 1
		REPS						
		WEIGHT						
		REPS						
		WEIGHT						
		REPS						
		WEIGHT						
		REPS						
		WEIGHT						
		REPS						
		WEIGHT						
		REPS						
		WEIGHT						
		REPS						
		WEIGHT						
		REPS						
		WEIGHT						

👟 CARDIO

EXERCISE	DURATION	DISTANCE	CALORIES	HEART RATE

NOTES / NUTRITION

RATING

⚡	BODY STRENGTH	☆☆☆☆☆
🧠	MIND POWER	☆☆☆☆☆

	DATE			TIME	
	WEIGHT			BODY FAT	
	MUSCLE GROUP		☐ WARM-UP		☐ STRETCH

STRENGTH TRAINING

EXERCISE			SET 1	SET 1	SET 1	SET 1	SET 1	SET 1
		REPS						
		WEIGHT						
		REPS						
		WEIGHT						
		REPS						
		WEIGHT						
		REPS						
		WEIGHT						
		REPS						
		WEIGHT						
		REPS						
		WEIGHT						
		REPS						
		WEIGHT						
		REPS						
		WEIGHT						

CARDIO

EXERCISE		DURATION	DISTANCE	CALORIES	HEART RATE

NOTES / NUTRITION

RATING

	BODY STRENGTH	☆☆☆☆☆
	MIND POWER	☆☆☆☆☆

📅 DATE		⏱ TIME	
⚖ WEIGHT		📏 BODY FAT	
💪 MUSCLE GROUP		☐ WARM-UP	☐ STRETCH

🏋 STRENGTH TRAINING			SET 1	SET 1	SET 1	SET 1	SET 1	SET 1
E X E R C I S E		REPS						
		WEIGHT						
		REPS						
		WEIGHT						
		REPS						
		WEIGHT						
		REPS						
		WEIGHT						
		REPS						
		WEIGHT						
		REPS						
		WEIGHT						
		REPS						
		WEIGHT						
		REPS						
		WEIGHT						

👟 CARDIO		DURATION	DISTANCE	CALORIES	HEART RATE
E X E R C I S E					

NOTES / NUTRITION

RATING	
⚡ BODY STRENGTH	☆☆☆☆☆
🧠 MIND POWER	☆☆☆☆☆

	DATE		TIME
	WEIGHT		BODY FAT
	MUSCLE GROUP	☐ WARM-UP	☐ STRETCH

STRENGTH TRAINING

EXERCISE			SET 1	SET 1	SET 1	SET 1	SET 1	SET 1
		REPS						
		WEIGHT						
		REPS						
		WEIGHT						
		REPS						
		WEIGHT						
		REPS						
		WEIGHT						
		REPS						
		WEIGHT						
		REPS						
		WEIGHT						
		REPS						
		WEIGHT						
		REPS						
		WEIGHT						

CARDIO

EXERCISE		DURATION	DISTANCE	CALORIES	HEART RATE

NOTES / NUTRITION

RATING

	BODY STRENGTH	☆☆☆☆☆
	MIND POWER	☆☆☆☆☆

	DATE		TIME
	WEIGHT		BODY FAT
	MUSCLE GROUP	☐ WARM-UP	☐ STRETCH

STRENGTH TRAINING

EXERCISE			SET 1	SET 1	SET 1	SET 1	SET 1	SET 1
		REPS						
		WEIGHT						
		REPS						
		WEIGHT						
		REPS						
		WEIGHT						
		REPS						
		WEIGHT						
		REPS						
		WEIGHT						
		REPS						
		WEIGHT						
		REPS						
		WEIGHT						
		REPS						
		WEIGHT						

CARDIO

EXERCISE		DURATION	DISTANCE	CALORIES	HEART RATE

NOTES / NUTRITION

RATING

⚡	BODY STRENGTH	☆☆☆☆☆
🧠	MIND POWER	☆☆☆☆☆

📅 DATE		⏱ TIME	
⚖ WEIGHT		📏 BODY FAT	
💪 MUSCLE GROUP		☐ WARM-UP	☐ STRETCH

🏋 STRENGTH TRAINING

			SET 1	SET 1	SET 1	SET 1	SET 1	SET 1
E X E R C I S E		REPS						
		WEIGHT						
		REPS						
		WEIGHT						
		REPS						
		WEIGHT						
		REPS						
		WEIGHT						
		REPS						
		WEIGHT						
		REPS						
		WEIGHT						
		REPS						
		WEIGHT						
		REPS						
		WEIGHT						

👟 CARDIO

		DURATION	DISTANCE	CALORIES	HEART RATE
E X E R C I S E					

NOTES / NUTRITION

RATING

⚡	BODY STRENGTH	☆☆☆☆☆
🧠	MIND POWER	☆☆☆☆☆

📅 DATE		🕐 TIME	
🪑 WEIGHT		📏 BODY FAT	
💪 MUSCLE GROUP		☐ WARM-UP	☐ STRETCH

🏋️ STRENGTH TRADING

STRENGTH TRAINING			SET 1	SET 1	SET 1	SET 1	SET 1	SET 1
EXERCISE		REPS						
		WEIGHT						
		REPS						
		WEIGHT						
		REPS						
		WEIGHT						
		REPS						
		WEIGHT						
		REPS						
		WEIGHT						
		REPS						
		WEIGHT						
		REPS						
		WEIGHT						
		REPS						
		WEIGHT						

👟 CARDIO

CARDIO		DURATION	DISTANCE	CALORIES	HEART RATE
EXERCISE					

NOTES / NUTRITION

RATING	
⚡ BODY STRENGTH	☆☆☆☆☆
🧠 MIND POWER	☆☆☆☆☆

📅 DATE		⏱️ TIME	
⚖️ WEIGHT		📏 BODY FAT	
💪 MUSCLE GROUP		☐ WARM-UP	☐ STRETCH

🏋️ STRENGTH TRAINING

EXERCISE			SET 1	SET 1	SET 1	SET 1	SET 1	SET 1
		REPS						
		WEIGHT						
		REPS						
		WEIGHT						
		REPS						
		WEIGHT						
		REPS						
		WEIGHT						
		REPS						
		WEIGHT						
		REPS						
		WEIGHT						
		REPS						
		WEIGHT						
		REPS						
		WEIGHT						

👟 CARDIO

EXERCISE		DURATION	DISTANCE	CALORIES	HEART RATE

NOTES / NUTRITION	RATING	
	⚡ BODY STRENGTH	☆☆☆☆☆
	🧠 MIND POWER	☆☆☆☆☆

📅 DATE		🕐 TIME	
⚖️ WEIGHT		📏 BODY FAT	
💪 MUSCLE GROUP		☐ WARM-UP	☐ STRETCH

🏋️ STRENGTH TRAINING			SET 1	SET 1	SET 1	SET 1	SET 1	SET 1
EXERCISE		REPS						
		WEIGHT						
		REPS						
		WEIGHT						
		REPS						
		WEIGHT						
		REPS						
		WEIGHT						
		REPS						
		WEIGHT						
		REPS						
		WEIGHT						
		REPS						
		WEIGHT						
		REPS						
		WEIGHT						

👟 CARDIO		DURATION	DISTANCE	CALORIES	HEART RATE
EXERCISE					

NOTES / NUTRITION

RATING	
⚡ BODY STRENGTH	☆☆☆☆☆
🧠 MIND POWER	☆☆☆☆☆

📅 DATE		⏱️ TIME	
🪣 WEIGHT		📏 BODY FAT	
💪 MUSCLE GROUP		☐ WARM-UP	☐ STRETCH

🏋️ STRENGTH TRAINING

EXERCISE			SET 1	SET 1	SET 1	SET 1	SET 1	SET 1
		REPS						
		WEIGHT						
		REPS						
		WEIGHT						
		REPS						
		WEIGHT						
		REPS						
		WEIGHT						
		REPS						
		WEIGHT						
		REPS						
		WEIGHT						
		REPS						
		WEIGHT						
		REPS						
		WEIGHT						

👟 CARDIO

EXERCISE		DURATION	DISTANCE	CALORIES	HEART RATE

NOTES / NUTRITION	RATING	
	⚡ BODY STRENGTH	☆☆☆☆☆
	🧠 MIND POWER	☆☆☆☆☆

📅 DATE		⏱️ TIME	
⚖️ WEIGHT		📏 BODY FAT	
💪 MUSCLE GROUP		☐ WARM-UP	☐ STRETCH

🏋️ STRENGTH TRAINING

EXERCISE			SET 1	SET 1	SET 1	SET 1	SET 1	SET 1
		REPS						
		WEIGHT						
		REPS						
		WEIGHT						
		REPS						
		WEIGHT						
		REPS						
		WEIGHT						
		REPS						
		WEIGHT						
		REPS						
		WEIGHT						
		REPS						
		WEIGHT						
		REPS						
		WEIGHT						

👟 CARDIO

EXERCISE		DURATION	DISTANCE	CALORIES	HEART RATE

NOTES / NUTRITION

RATING

⚡	BODY STRENGTH	☆☆☆☆☆
🧠	MIND POWER	☆☆☆☆☆

www.ingramcontent.com/pod-product-compliance
Lightning Source LLC
Chambersburg PA
CBHW080600030426
42336CB00019B/3271